AFIB DIET

COOKBOOK FOR

BEGINNERS

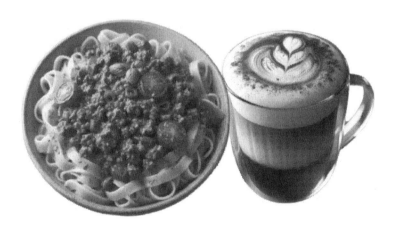

Heart-Healthy Recipes to Regulate Arrhythmia
and Lower Blood Pressure

Lanita Cruz

Copyright © 2024 by Lanita Cruz

Table of Contents

Disclaimer

The information provided in this cookbook is for educational and informational purposes only. It is not intended to be a substitute for professional medical advice, diagnosis, or treatment.

Always seek the advice of your physician or other qualified health provider with any questions you may have regarding a medical condition.

The recipes and dietary suggestions included are based on general principles and may not be suitable for everyone.

Individual dietary needs and health conditions vary, and it is essential to consult with a healthcare professional before making significant changes to your diet.

The author and publisher disclaim responsibility for any effects resulting directly or indirectly from the use or misuse of the information provided in this cookbook.

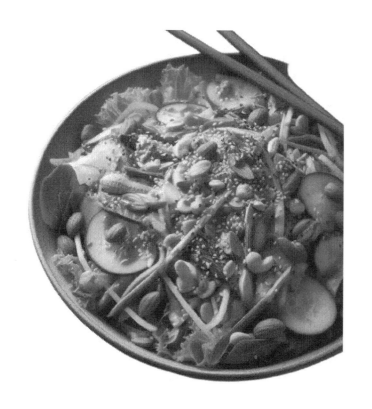

Introduction

Have you ever felt overwhelmed by the abundance of dietary advice for managing atrial fibrillation? Are you seeking not just a meal plan, but a lifestyle change that harmonizes with your heart's rhythm?

If these questions resonate with you, you're in the right place. This Afib cookbook is more than a collection of recipes; it's a beacon of hope and a testament to the healing power of food.

In this book, together you and I will delve into the core principles of the Afib Diet, uncover the myriad benefits it offers, and I will equip you with practical insights on the foods to embrace and those to avoid.

Understanding the intricate relationship between nutrition and atrial fibrillation is important, and that's precisely where our journey begins.

From exploring the foods that grace your plate to deciphering the ones best left aside, we'll navigate the dietary landscape with clarity and purpose. The comprehensive shopping list provided will be your ally in creating a heart-healthy pantry that supports your commitment to wellness.

In the recipe sections of this book, you'll embark on a culinary journey designed to support your cardiac health. You'll discover dishes that are not only delectable but also tailored to reduce inflammation, balance electrolytes, and provide the nutrients essential for a steady heartbeat.

From vibrant breakfast options to satisfying dinners and tempting but healthy desserts and snacks. Each recipe is carefully crafted to not only meet the requirements of the Afib Diet but to tantalize your taste buds and make healthy eating an enjoyable, flavorful experience

What sets this book apart is its commitment to scientific evidence and practicality, ensuring that each recipe is both beneficial and achievable.

You're not alone on this path. Countless others share your quest for a heart-healthy diet that doesn't sacrifice flavor or joy. Together, we'll explore the synergy between taste and well-being, proving that food can be both medicine and pleasure.

As you turn the pages, you'll find yourself equipped with the knowledge to make informed choices, the inspiration to continue your journey, and the confidence to take control of your health.

As we journey through these pages, you'll also find a 30-day meal plan sample, offering a practical guide to seamlessly incorporate Afib-friendly meals into your daily life.

So, whether you're a newcomer to the Afib Diet or a seasoned practitioner looking for fresh inspiration, let's embark on this gastronomic adventure that nourishes your heart, body, and soul.

Are you ready? Turn to the next page where we begin with "Principles of the Afib Diet" Get ready to savor the joy of heart-healthy living—one delicious recipe at a time.

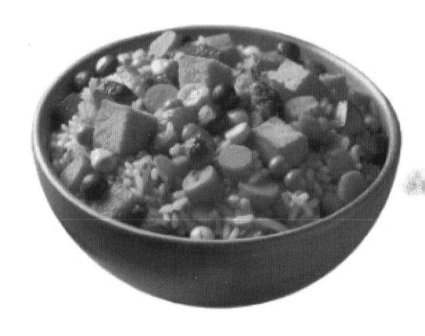

CHAPTER 1

Principles of the Afib Diet

The Afib diet is a dietary approach that aims to reduce the risk of atrial fibrillation, a common heart rhythm disorder that can cause strokes, heart failure, and other complications. The Afib diet is based on the following principles:

- Eat more plant-based foods, such as fruits, vegetables, whole grains, nuts, seeds, and legumes. These foods are rich in fiber, antioxidants, and anti-inflammatory compounds that can help lower blood pressure, cholesterol, and inflammation, which are all risk factors for atrial fibrillation .

- Limit animal-based foods, especially red meat, processed meat, and dairy products. These foods are high in saturated fat, cholesterol, and sodium, which can increase blood pressure, cholesterol, and inflammation, as well as trigger arrhythmias.

- Avoid foods and drinks that contain caffeine, alcohol, or added sugar. These substances can stimulate the heart and cause irregular heartbeats, as well as increase blood pressure, cholesterol, and inflammation.
- Choose healthy fats, like avocado, olive oil, and fatty fish. These fats are rich in monounsaturated and omega-3 fatty acids, which can improve heart health, lower inflammation, and prevent blood clots.
- Stay hydrated and limit salt intake. Drinking enough water can help prevent dehydration, which can trigger arrhythmias, as well as flush out excess sodium and toxins from the body . Limiting salt intake can help lower blood pressure and fluid retention, which can strain the heart .

By following these principles, the Afib diet can help you manage your condition, prevent complications, and improve your overall health and well-being.

Benefits of the Afib Diet

1. Heart Rhythm Harmony:

A primary benefit of the Afib Diet is its positive impact on heart rhythm. By prioritizing nutrient-dense foods and steering clear of potential triggers, individuals may experience a more stable and regular heartbeat, contributing to improved overall cardiovascular health.

2. Inflammation Reduction:

The Afib Diet's emphasis on omega-3 fatty acids and anti-inflammatory foods serves as a powerful tool in reducing inflammation. This, in turn, may mitigate the risk factors associated with atrial fibrillation, fostering a heart environment that thrives on balance.

3. Blood Pressure Regulation:

The principles of the Afib Diet align with strategies for maintaining healthy blood pressure levels. Through the incorporation of heart-healthy foods and mindful sodium moderation, individuals may experience improved blood pressure regulation, a critical factor in heart health.

4. Nutrient-Packed Wellness:

By focusing on whole, nutrient-dense foods, the Afib Diet becomes a source of comprehensive wellness. Essential vitamins, minerals, and antioxidants abundant in fruits, vegetables, and lean proteins contribute to overall health, providing the body with the tools it needs to function optimally.

5. Weight Management:

A natural outcome of adopting the Afib Diet is often weight management. With an emphasis on balanced nutrition and portion control, individuals may find it easier to achieve and maintain a healthy weight. This, in turn, positively impacts cardiovascular health and reduces the strain on the heart.

6. Sustainable Energy Levels:

The Afib Diet isn't just about what you avoid; it's about embracing foods that fuel sustainable energy levels. By choosing complex carbohydrates, lean proteins, and heart-healthy fats, individuals may experience sustained energy throughout the day, supporting both physical and cardiovascular activities.

7. Holistic Well-Being:

Beyond the physical benefits, the Afib Diet promotes holistic well-being. The psychological satisfaction derived from enjoying delicious, heart-healthy meals contributes to a positive mindset, creating a harmonious balance between nourishing the body and delighting the senses.

Foods to Eat

1. Lean Proteins:

Incorporate lean protein sources such as skinless poultry, fish, tofu, and legumes. These provide essential amino acids without the saturated fat content often found in red meats.

2. Colorful Fruits and Vegetables:

Fill your plate with a vibrant array of fruits and vegetables. These nutritional powerhouses are rich in antioxidants, vitamins, and minerals, contributing to heart health and overall well-being.

3. Whole Grains:

Choose whole grains like brown rice, quinoa, and oats. These grains offer fiber, promote digestive health, and provide a steady release of energy, supporting sustained daily activities.

4. Fatty Fish:

Integrate fatty fish, such as salmon, mackerel, and trout, into your diet. Packed with omega-3 fatty acids, these fish contribute to heart health by reducing inflammation and supporting optimal heart rhythm.

5. Nuts and Seeds:

Enjoy a variety of nuts and seeds, such as almonds, walnuts, chia seeds, and flaxseeds. These are excellent sources of heart-healthy fats, fiber, and essential nutrients.

6. Dairy or Dairy Alternatives:

Include low-fat dairy or fortified dairy alternatives in your diet. These provide calcium and vitamin D, essential for bone health and overall well-being.

7. Olive Oil:

Choose olive oil as your primary cooking oil. Rich in monounsaturated fats, olive oil supports heart health and adds a delightful flavor to your dishes.

8. Avocados:

Indulge in the creamy goodness of avocados. Packed with monounsaturated fats, potassium, and fiber, avocados contribute to heart health and satiety.

Foods to Avoid

1. Excessive Sodium:

Limit your intake of high-sodium foods, as excess sodium can contribute to elevated blood pressure. Be cautious with processed foods, canned soups, and salty snacks.

2. Saturated and Trans Fats:

Steer clear of saturated and trans fats found in fried foods, processed snacks, and certain baked goods. These fats can increase cholesterol levels and pose risks to heart health.

3. Added Sugars:

Minimize your consumption of added sugars. Watch out for sugary beverages, candies, and processed foods, as excessive sugar intake can contribute to inflammation and other cardiovascular issues.

4. Caffeine and Stimulants:

While moderate caffeine intake is generally acceptable, excessive consumption may trigger atrial fibrillation episodes in some individuals. Be mindful of your caffeine sources and consider moderation.

5. Alcohol in Excess:

Limit alcohol intake, as excessive alcohol consumption can disrupt heart rhythm and contribute to atrial fibrillation. It is better to not drink at all, but if you decide to drink, do so in moderation, adhering to recommended guidelines.

6. High Oxalate Foods:

For individuals sensitive to oxalates, limit high-oxalate foods like spinach, beets, and nuts. Oxalates can contribute to the formation of kidney stones, which may exacerbate health issues.

7. Processed Meats:

Reduce your intake of processed meats, as they often contain high levels of sodium and unhealthy fats. Choose leaner protein sources like fish, poultry, or plant-based alternatives.

8. Trigger Foods:

Identify and avoid specific trigger foods that may exacerbate atrial fibrillation symptoms for some individuals. This can include items like spicy foods, chocolate, or certain food additives.

Comprehensive Shopping List for Afib Diet

Proteins:
- Skinless poultry (chicken, turkey)
- Fatty fish (salmon, mackerel, trout)
- Tofu and tempeh
- Legumes (lentils, chickpeas, black beans)

Fruits and Vegetables:

- Leafy greens (spinach, kale, Swiss chard)
- Colorful bell peppers
- Berries (blueberries, strawberries, raspberries)
- Avocados
- Broccoli and cauliflower
- Sweet potatoes
- Citrus fruits (oranges, grapefruits)

Whole Grains:

- Quinoa
- Brown rice
- Oats
- Whole wheat pasta
- Barley

Nuts and Seeds:

- Almonds
- Walnuts
- Chia seeds
- Flaxseeds
- Sunflower seeds

Dairy or Dairy Alternatives:

- Low-fat yogurt
- Skim milk
- Fortified almond or soy milk
- Cheese in moderation

Oils and Fats:

- Olive oil
- Avocado oil
- Nuts and seeds (in moderation)

Herbs and Spices:

- Turmeric
- Ginger
- Garlic
- Cinnamon
- Basil
- Rosemary

Beverages:

- Water (stay hydrated)
- Herbal teas (caffeine-free options)

- Limited caffeine-containing beverages (if tolerated)

Miscellaneous:
- Honey or maple syrup (as natural sweeteners)
- Whole-grain or multigrain bread
- Eggs
- Dark chocolate (in moderation)

Fresh Produce (as per seasonal availability):
- Tomatoes
- Cucumbers
- Zucchini
- Berries
- Apples
- Grapes

CHAPTER 2

Delicious and Nutritious Recipes for Afib Diet

Breakfast Recipes for Afib Diet

Peanut Butter-Banana Cinnamon Toast

- Preparation Time: 5 minutes
- Serves: 1

Ingredients:

- 1 slice whole-grain bread
- 1 tablespoon natural peanut butter
- 1/2 banana, sliced
- 1/4 teaspoon ground cinnamon
- Drizzle of honey (optional)

Nutritional Information: Calories: 280 | Protein: 8g | Fat: 13g | Carbohydrates: 35g | Fiber: 6g | Sugars: 11g

Instructions:

1. Toast the whole-grain bread slice to your liking.

2. Spread the natural peanut butter evenly on the toasted bread.
3. Spread the banana slices evenly over the peanut butter.
4. Sprinkle ground cinnamon over the banana slices.
5. For added sweetness, drizzle honey over the toast if desired.

Serving Suggestions:

Enjoy this delightful Peanut Butter-Banana Cinnamon Toast as a quick and nutritious breakfast alongside a cup of herbal tea or your favorite heart-healthy beverage.

Mango-Almond Smoothie Bowl

- **Preparation Time:** 10 minutes
- **Serves: 1**

Ingredients:

- 1 cup frozen mango chunks
- 1/2 ripe banana
- 1/2 cup almond milk
- 1/4 cup rolled oats

- 1 tablespoon almond butter
- Toppings: Sliced almonds, chia seeds, fresh mango chunks

Nutritional Information: Calories: 380 | Protein: 8g | Fat: 15g | Carbohydrates: 58g | Fiber: 9g | Sugars: 28g

Instructions:

1. In a blender, combine frozen mango chunks, banana, almond milk, rolled oats, and almond butter.
2. Blend until smooth and creamy.
3. Pour the smoothie into a bowl.
4. Top with sliced almonds, chia seeds, and fresh mango chunks.

Serving Suggestions:

Indulge in the Mango-Almond Smoothie Bowl for a refreshing and nutrient-packed breakfast. Customize with additional toppings such as granola or shredded coconut for added texture.

Vegan Breakfast Burrito

- **Preparation Time:** 15 minutes
- **Serves:** 2

Ingredients:

- 1 cup firm tofu, crumbled
- 1 tablespoon olive oil
- 1/2 bell pepper, diced
- 1/2 onion, diced
- 1 clove garlic, minced
- 1 teaspoon ground cumin
- 1/2 teaspoon turmeric powder
- Salt and pepper to taste
- 4 whole-grain tortillas
- Salsa and avocado for topping

Nutritional Information: Calories: 320 | Protein: 15g | Fat: 14g | Carbohydrates: 36g | Fiber: 8g | Sugars: 4g

Instructions:

1. In a skillet, sauté diced bell pepper, onion, and minced garlic in olive oil until softened.
2. Add crumbled tofu to the skillet and cook until heated through.
3. Sprinkle ground cumin, turmeric powder, salt, and pepper over the tofu mixture. Stir well.
4. Warm the whole-grain tortillas in a separate pan or microwave.
5. Spoon the tofu mixture onto each tortilla.
6. Top with salsa and sliced avocado.
7. Fold the tortillas to form burritos.

Serving Suggestions: Serve the Vegan Breakfast Burritos with a side of fresh fruit or a green salad for a satisfying and plant-based breakfast.

Almond Flour Banana Bread

- **Preparation Time:** 15 minutes
- **Baking Time:** 45-50 minutes
- **Serves:** 8 slices

Ingredients:
- 2 ripe bananas, mashed

- 3 large eggs
- 1/4 cup coconut oil, melted
- 1/4 cup almond milk
- 1 teaspoon vanilla extract
- 2 cups almond flour
- 1 teaspoon baking powder
- 1/2 teaspoon baking soda
- 1/4 teaspoon salt
- 1 teaspoon ground cinnamon
- 1/2 cup chopped walnuts (optional)

Nutritional Information: Calories: 210 | Protein: 7g | Fat: 18g | Carbohydrates: 10g | Fiber: 3g | Sugars: 4g

Instructions:

1. Preheat the oven to 350°F (175°C). Grease a loaf pan.
2. In a large bowl, mash the ripe bananas.
3. Add eggs, melted coconut oil, almond milk, and vanilla extract. Mix well.
4. In a separate bowl, combine almond flour, baking powder, baking soda, salt, and ground cinnamon.

5. Add the dry ingredients gradually to the banana mixture, stirring continuously until fully integrated.
6. If desired, fold in chopped walnuts.
7. Fill the prepared loaf pan with the batter.
8. Allow the bread to bake for 45-50 minutes until a toothpick inserted into the center comes out clean.
9. Let your banana bread cool before slicing.

Serving Suggestions: Enjoy a slice of Almond Flour Banana Bread with a dollop of Greek yogurt or spread with natural almond butter for added protein and flavor.

Mediterranean Breakfast Salad

- **Preparation Time:** 10 minutes
- **Serves:** 2

Ingredients:

- 2 cups of mixed greens (arugula, spinach, or kale)
- 1 cup cherry tomatoes, halved

- 1/2 cucumber, sliced
- 1/4 cup Kalamata olives, pitted
- 1/4 cup feta cheese, crumbled
- 2 poached eggs
- 2 tablespoons extra-virgin olive oil
- 1 tablespoon balsamic vinegar
- Salt and pepper to taste
- Fresh basil leaves for garnish

Nutritional Information: Calories: 280 | Protein: 12g | Fat: 21g | Carbohydrates: 15g | Fiber: 5g | Sugars: 7g

Instructions:

1. In a large bowl, combine mixed greens, cherry tomatoes, cucumber, Kalamata olives, and feta cheese.
2. In a separate pan, poach two eggs until the whites are set but the yolks are still runny.
3. Place the poached eggs on top of the salad.
4. Drizzle your salad with balsamic vinegar and extra-virgin olive oil.
5. Season with salt and pepper to suit your liking.

6. Garnish with fresh basil leaves.

Serving Suggestions: Serve the Mediterranean Breakfast Salad with a slice of whole-grain bread or a side of quinoa for a complete and satisfying morning meal.

Creamy Blueberry-Pecan Oatmeal

- **Preparation Time:** 10 minutes
- **Serves:** 2

Ingredients:

- 1 cup old-fashioned oats
- 2 cups almond milk
- 1 cup fresh or frozen blueberries
- 1/4 cup chopped pecans
- 1 tablespoon chia seeds
- 1 tablespoon maple syrup
- 1/2 teaspoon vanilla extract
- Pinch of salt
- Fresh blueberries and pecans for topping

Nutritional Information: Calories: 350 | Protein: 9g | Fat: 14g | Carbohydrates: 50g | Fiber: 10g | Sugars: 15g

Instructions:

1. In a saucepan, combine old-fashioned oats, almond milk, blueberries, chopped pecans, chia seeds, maple syrup, vanilla extract, and a pinch of salt.
2. Bring the mixture to a gentle simmer on medium heat.
3. Cook, stirring occasionally, for 5-7 minutes or until the oats are tender and the blueberries burst.
4. Remove it from the heat and allow it to sit for a couple of minutes to thicken.
5. Divide the creamy oatmeal into bowls.
6. Top with fresh blueberries and additional chopped pecans.

Serving Suggestions: Serve this Creamy Blueberry-Pecan Oatmeal with a dollop of Greek yogurt or a splash of almond milk for added creaminess and protein.

Banana Nut Pancakes

- **Preparation Time:** 15 minutes
- **Cooking Time:** 10 minutes
- **Serves:** 2

Ingredients:

- 1 cup whole wheat flour
- 1 tablespoon baking powder
- 1/4 teaspoon salt
- 1 ripe banana, mashed
- 1 cup almond milk
- 1 tablespoon coconut oil, melted
- 1/4 cup chopped walnuts
- Maple syrup for drizzling

Nutritional Information: Calories: 320 | Protein: 8g | Fat: 14g | Carbohydrates: 40g | Fiber: 7g | Sugars: 8g

Instructions:

1. In a large bowl, whisk together whole wheat flour, baking powder, and salt.
2. In a separate bowl, mix mashed banana, almond milk, and melted coconut oil.
3. Stir the wet mixture into the dry ingredients until blended.
4. Fold in chopped walnuts.
5. Heat up a griddle or non-stick skillet at medium temperature.
6. Portion out 1/4 cup of batter onto the griddle to make each pancake.
7. Cook until bubbles appear on the surface, then flip and continue cooking until golden brown.
8. Arrange the pancakes in a stack and pour maple syrup over them.

Serving Suggestions: Pair these Banana Nut Pancakes with a side of fresh fruit or a small serving of Greek yogurt for a delightful and satisfying breakfast.

Lunch Recipes for Afib Diet

Soft Scrambled Tofu with Veggies

- **Preparation Time:** 15 minutes
- **Cooking Time:** 10 minutes
- **Serves:** 2

Ingredients:

- 1 block (14 oz) of drained and crumbled extra-firm tofu
- 1 tablespoon olive oil
- 1/2 onion, diced
- 1 bell pepper, diced
- 1 cup spinach leaves
- 2 cloves garlic, minced
- 1/2 teaspoon ground turmeric
- Salt and pepper to taste
- Fresh parsley for garnish (optional)

Nutritional Information (per serving): Calories: 180 | Protein: 12g | Fat: 10g | Carbohydrates: 10g | Fiber: 3g | Sugars: 3g

Instructions:

1. In a large skillet, heat your olive oil over medium heat until warm.
2. Add diced onion and bell pepper to the skillet. Cook until softened, about 3-4 minutes.
3. Add minced garlic and cook for another 1-2 minutes until fragrant.
4. Add your ground turmeric and crumbled tofu to the skillet. Stir well to combine.
5. Cook for 5-6 minutes, stirring occasionally, until the tofu is heated through and slightly golden.
6. Stir in spinach leaves and cook until wilted.
7. Season with salt and pepper to suit your liking.
8. Garnish with fresh parsley if desired.

Serving Suggestions: Serve the Soft Scrambled Tofu with Veggies hot, alongside whole-grain toast or a side salad for a nutritious and satisfying lunch.

Garlic Mashed Cauliflower

- **Preparation Time:** 10 minutes
- **Cooking Time:** 15 minutes
- **Serves:** 4

Ingredients:

- 1 head cauliflower, cut into florets
- 2 cloves garlic, minced
- 2 tablespoons olive oil
- 1/4 cup unsweetened almond milk
- Salt and pepper to taste
- Fresh chives for garnish (optional)

Nutritional Information (per serving): Calories: 80 | Protein: 2g | Fat: 5g | Carbohydrates: 8g | Fiber: 3g | Sugars: 3g

Instructions:

1. Steam or boil cauliflower florets until tender, about 8-10 minutes.
2. Get a skillet and heat your olive oil over medium heat.

3. Place minced garlic in the skillet, cooking until fragrant, usually 1-2 minutes.
4. Transfer the cooked cauliflower to a food processor after draining.
5. Add the sautéed garlic, olive oil, and almond milk to the food processor.
6. Blend until smooth and creamy.
7. Season with salt and pepper to suit your liking.
8. Garnish with fresh chives if desired.

Serving Suggestions: Enjoy the Garlic Mashed Cauliflower as a delicious and nutritious side dish alongside grilled chicken or fish, or as a creamy base for roasted vegetables.

Lemon Rosemary Chicken

- **Preparation Time:** 10 minutes
- **Marinating Time:** 30 minutes (optional)
- **Cooking Time:** 20 minutes
- **Serves:** 2

Ingredients:

- 2 boneless, skinless chicken breasts
- 2 tablespoons olive oil

- 2 cloves garlic, minced
- 1 lemon, juiced and zested
- 1 tablespoon fresh rosemary, chopped
- Salt and pepper to taste
- Lemon slices for garnish (optional)
- Fresh rosemary sprigs for garnish (optional)

Nutritional Information (per serving): Calories: 250 | Protein: 25g | Fat: 14g | Carbohydrates: 4g | Fiber: 1g | Sugars: 1g

Instructions:

1. In a bowl, whisk together olive oil, minced garlic, lemon juice, lemon zest, chopped rosemary, salt, and pepper.
2. Put the chicken breasts in a resealable plastic bag or shallow dish.
3. Make sure the chicken is coated by pouring the marinade evenly over it.
4. Marinate in the refrigerator for at least 30 minutes, if time allows.
5. Preheat your grill or grill pan to medium-high heat.

6. Remove the chicken from the marinade, discarding any leftover marinade.
7. Grill the chicken until it's fully cooked, about 6-8 minutes on each side.
8. Take the chicken off the grill and allow it to rest for a few moments before serving.
9. Garnish with lemon slices and fresh rosemary sprigs if desired.

Serving Suggestions: Serve the Lemon Rosemary Chicken with a side of steamed vegetables or a mixed green salad for a flavorful and protein-packed lunch.

Spring Vegetable Stir-Fried Rice

- **Preparation Time:** 10 minutes
- **Cooking Time:** 15 minutes
- **Serves:** 4

Ingredients:
- 2 cups cooked brown rice, chilled
- 1 tablespoon sesame oil
- 2 cloves garlic, minced
- 1 cup asparagus spears, trimmed and cut into pieces

- 1 cup snap peas, trimmed
- 1 small red bell pepper, diced
- 1 small carrot, julienned
- 2 green onions, thinly sliced
- 2 tablespoons low-sodium soy sauce
- 1 tablespoon rice vinegar
- 1 teaspoon honey or maple syrup
- 1 teaspoon grated ginger
- Sesame seeds for garnish (optional)

Nutritional Information (per serving): Calories: 220 | Protein: 6g | Fat: 5g | Carbohydrates: 38g | Fiber: 5g | Sugars: 6g

Instructions:

1. Warm sesame oil in a large skillet or wok, maintaining medium heat.
2. Add minced garlic to the skillet and sauté for 1 minute until fragrant.
3. Add asparagus, snap peas, red bell pepper, and carrot to the skillet. Stir-fry the vegetables until they are tender-crisp, about 3-4 minutes.

4. Add chilled cooked brown rice to the skillet. Stir-fry for another 3-4 minutes until heated through.

5. Whisk together low-sodium soy sauce, rice vinegar, honey, or maple syrup, and grated ginger in a small bowl until thoroughly mixed.

6. Pour the sauce over the rice and vegetables in the skillet. Stir well to coat evenly.

7. Cook for another 1-2 minutes until the sauce is heated through and everything is well combined.

8. Take the pan off the heat and sprinkle sliced green onions and sesame seeds on top, if you like.

Serving Suggestions: Serve the Spring Vegetable Stir-Fried Rice as a wholesome and colorful lunch option, garnished with extra sliced green onions and a sprinkle of sesame seeds for added flavor and texture.

Easy Tofu Fajitas (Vegan)

- **Preparation Time:** 10 minutes
- **Cooking Time:** 15 minutes
- **Serves:** 4

Ingredients:

- 1 block (14 oz) of drained and pressed firm tofu
- 2 bell peppers, sliced
- 1 onion, sliced
- 2 tablespoons olive oil
- 2 cloves garlic, minced
- 1 tablespoon chili powder
- 1 teaspoon ground cumin
- 1 teaspoon smoked paprika
- Salt and pepper to taste
- 8 small whole-grain tortillas
- Optional toppings: Sliced avocado, salsa, chopped cilantro, lime wedges

Nutritional Information (per serving): Calories: 240 | Protein: 10g | Fat: 10g | Carbohydrates: 30g | Fiber: 7g | Sugars: 5g

Instructions:

1. Slice the pressed tofu into thin strips.

2. In a large skillet, heat your olive oil over medium heat.

3. Place sliced bell peppers and onions in the skillet. Sauté until softened, about 5-6 minutes.

4. Add minced garlic, chili powder, ground cumin, smoked paprika, salt, and pepper to the skillet. Stir well to coat the vegetables with the spices.

5. Push the vegetables to one side of the skillet and add the tofu strips to the empty side.

6. Cook the tofu for 3-4 minutes on each side until lightly browned and heated through.

7. Warm the whole-grain tortillas in a separate pan or microwave.

8. Serve the tofu and vegetable mixture in the warm tortillas.

9. Garnish with sliced avocado, salsa, chopped cilantro, and lime wedges if desired.

Serving Suggestions: Enjoy these Easy Tofu Fajitas with your favorite toppings for a flavorful and satisfying vegan lunch option. Serve alongside a side salad or brown rice for a complete meal.

Colorful Veggie Stew with Turkey Tenders

- **Preparation Time:** 15 minutes
- **Cooking Time:** 25 minutes
- **Serves:** 4

Ingredients:

- 1 lb turkey breast tenders, cut into bite-sized pieces
- 1 tablespoon olive oil
- 1 onion, diced
- 2 cloves garlic, minced
- 2 carrots, diced
- 2 celery stalks, diced
- 1 bell pepper, diced
- 1 zucchini, diced
- 1 can (14 oz) diced tomatoes, undrained
- 4 cups low-sodium vegetable broth
- 1 teaspoon dried thyme
- 1 teaspoon dried oregano
- Salt and pepper to taste
- Fresh parsley for garnish (optional)

Nutritional Information (per serving): Calories: 280 | Protein: 28g | Fat: 6g | Carbohydrates: 28g | Fiber: 7g | Sugars: 12g

Instructions:

1. Heat your olive oil in a large pot over medium heat.
2. Add diced onion and minced garlic to the pot. Sauté for 2-3 minutes until fragrant.
3. Add turkey breast tenders to the pot. Cook until uniformly browned, roughly 5 minutes in total.
4. Add diced carrots, celery, bell pepper, and zucchini to the pot. Cook for another 5 minutes until vegetables begin to soften.
5. Pour in diced tomatoes (with their juices) and low-sodium vegetable broth.
6. Stir in dried thyme and dried oregano. Season with salt and pepper to suit your liking.
7. Bring the stew to a simmer and let it cook for 15-20 minutes until the vegetables are tender and the turkey is cooked through.

8. Remove from heat and ladle the stew into bowls.

9. Garnish with fresh parsley if desired.

Serving Suggestions: Serve the Colorful Veggie Stew with Turkey Tenders hot, with a side of whole-grain bread or a simple green salad for a nutritious and satisfying lunch.

Raw Vegan Gazpacho

- **Preparation Time:** 15 minutes
- **Chilling Time:** 2 hours
- **Serves:** 4

Ingredients:

- 4 large tomatoes, diced
- 1 cucumber, peeled and diced
- 1 red bell pepper, diced
- 1/2 red onion, diced
- 2 cloves garlic, minced
- 2 tablespoons extra-virgin olive oil
- 2 tablespoons red wine vinegar
- 1 tablespoon fresh lemon juice

- 1 teaspoon dried oregano
- Salt and pepper to taste
- 1 cup vegetable broth (optional, for a thinner consistency)
- Fresh basil leaves for garnish (optional)

Nutritional Information (per serving): Calories: 120 | Protein: 2g | Fat: 7g | Carbohydrates: 14g | Fiber: 4g | Sugars: 7g

Instructions:

1. In a blender or food processor, combine diced tomatoes, cucumber, red bell pepper, red onion, minced garlic, extra-virgin olive oil, red wine vinegar, fresh lemon juice, dried oregano, salt, and pepper.
2. Blend until smooth and well combined. If a thinner consistency is desired, add vegetable broth and blend again.
3. Pour the gazpacho into a bowl or pitcher for serving.
4. Cover and refrigerate for at least 2 hours to chill.

5. Before serving, taste and adjust seasoning if necessary.
6. Ladle the chilled gazpacho into bowls.
7. Garnish with fresh basil leaves if desired.

Serving Suggestions: Serve the Raw Vegan Gazpacho cold, garnished with fresh basil leaves and a drizzle of extra-virgin olive oil. Pair with a slice of whole-grain bread or a side of mixed greens for a light and refreshing lunch option.

Dinner Recipes for Afib

Mexican Platter

- **Preparation Time:** 20 minutes
- **Cooking Time:** 20 minutes
- **Serves:** 4

Ingredients:

- 1 cup cooked quinoa
- 1 cup black beans, rinsed and drained
- 1 cup corn kernels (fresh or frozen)
- 1 avocado, sliced

- 1 cup cherry tomatoes, halved
- 1/2 red onion, thinly sliced
- 1 jalapeño, thinly sliced (optional)
- Fresh cilantro leaves for garnish
- Lime wedges for serving

For the Salsa:

- 2 tomatoes, diced
- 1/2 red onion, finely chopped
- 1/4 cup chopped fresh cilantro
- 1 jalapeño, seeded and minced
- Juice of 1 lime
- Salt and pepper to taste

For the Guacamole:

- 2 ripe avocados
- 1/4 cup diced red onion
- 1/4 cup chopped fresh cilantro
- Juice of 1 lime
- Salt and pepper to taste

Nutritional Information (per serving): Calories: 320 | Protein: 10g | Fat: 15g | Carbohydrates: 40g | Fiber: 12g | Sugars: 4g

Instructions:

1. Follow the package directions to cook quinoa and then set it aside.
2. In a bowl, combine diced tomatoes, chopped red onion, chopped cilantro, minced jalapeño (if using), lime juice, salt, and pepper to make the salsa. Set aside.
3. In another bowl, mash ripe avocados and mix with diced red onion, chopped cilantro, lime juice, salt, and pepper to make the guacamole. Set aside.
4. In a skillet, heat black beans and corn kernels until heated through.
5. Arrange cooked quinoa, black beans, corn, sliced avocado, cherry tomatoes, red onion, and jalapeño (if using) on a large platter.
6. Garnish with fresh cilantro leaves.

7. Serve with lime wedges, salsa, and guacamole on the side.

Serving Suggestions: Serve the Mexican Platter as a build-your-own meal, allowing each person to assemble their own bowls or tacos using the various components. Enjoy with whole-grain tortillas or lettuce wraps for a nutritious and flavorful dinner option.

Egg Drop Soup

- **Preparation Time:** 10 minutes
- **Cooking Time:** 10 minutes
- **Serves:** 2

Ingredients:

- 4 cups low-sodium chicken or vegetable broth
- 2 large eggs, lightly beaten
- 1 tablespoon soy sauce
- 1 teaspoon sesame oil
- 2 green onions, thinly sliced
- Salt and pepper to taste
- Fresh cilantro leaves for garnish (optional)

Nutritional Information (per serving): Calories: 80 | Protein: 7g | Fat: 4g | Carbohydrates: 3g | Fiber: 0g | Sugars: 1g

Instructions:

1. Heat the chicken or vegetable broth in a saucepan until it simmers over medium heat.
2. While stirring the broth gently, slowly pour in the beaten eggs in a steady stream.
3. Let the eggs cook for a few seconds until they form thin ribbons.
4. Stir in soy sauce and sesame oil.
5. Season with salt and pepper to suit your liking.
6. Remove from heat and garnish with thinly sliced green onions and fresh cilantro leaves if desired.
7. Serve hot.

Serving Suggestions: Enjoy the Egg Drop Soup as a light and comforting dinner option. Pair with a side of steamed vegetables or a small salad for added nutrition.

Rainbow Collard Wraps

- **Preparation Time:** 15 minutes
- **Serves:** 4

Ingredients:

- 8 large collard green leaves
- 1 cup cooked quinoa or brown rice
- 1 cup shredded carrots
- 1 cup thinly sliced red cabbage
- 1 bell pepper, thinly sliced
- 1 avocado, sliced
- Hummus or tahini for spreading
- Fresh cilantro leaves for garnish (optional)

Nutritional Information (per serving, with quinoa):
Calories: 180 | Protein: 5g | Fat: 8g | Carbohydrates: 25g | Fiber: 8g | Sugars: 4g

Instructions:
1. Wash the collard green leaves and pat them dry with paper towels.
2. Trim the thick stem from each collard green leaf to make it easier to roll.

3. Lay a collard green leaf flat on a clean surface.
4. Spread a thin layer of hummus or tahini onto the center of the leaf.
5. Layer cooked quinoa or brown rice, shredded carrots, sliced red cabbage, bell pepper, and avocado slices on top of the hummus.
6. Fold the sides of the collard green leaf inward, then roll it up tightly like a burrito.
7. Fill and roll up the remaining collard green leaves using the same method.
8. Slice each wrap in half diagonally.
9. Serve immediately, garnished with fresh cilantro leaves if desired.

Serving Suggestions: Enjoy the Rainbow Collard Wraps as a vibrant and nutritious dinner option. Pair with a side of roasted sweet potatoes or a mixed green salad for a complete meal.

Ginger Carrot Soup

- **Preparation Time:** 10 minutes
- **Cooking Time:** 25 minutes
- **Serves:** 4

Ingredients:

- 1 tablespoon olive oil
- 1 onion, chopped
- 3 cloves garlic, minced
- 1 tablespoon fresh ginger, grated
- 6 large carrots, peeled and chopped
- 4 cups low-sodium vegetable broth
- 1 teaspoon ground turmeric
- Salt and pepper to taste
- 1/4 cup coconut milk (optional, for garnish)
- Fresh cilantro leaves for garnish (optional)

Nutritional Information (per serving): Calories: 120 | Protein: 2g | Fat: 4g | Carbohydrates: 20g | Fiber: 5g | Sugars: 10g

Instructions:

1. In a large pot, heat olive oil over medium heat.

2. Add your chopped onion and sauté it until translucent, should take 5 minutes.

3. Add your minced garlic and grated ginger to the pot. Stir and cook for an extra 1-2 minutes to enhance the scent.

4. Add chopped carrots to the pot and stir well to combine.

5. Add low-sodium vegetable broth to the pot and bring it to a boil.

6. Reduce heat to low and simmer for 15-20 minutes until the carrots are tender.

7. Puree the soup with an immersion blender until it reaches a smooth consistency.

8. You can also blend the soup in batches using a blender until smooth, and then transfer it back into the pot.

9. Stir in ground turmeric and Season with salt and pepper to suit your liking.

10. If desired, swirl in coconut milk for added creaminess.

11. For extra freshness and appeal, serve the dish hot, and if desired, sprinkle with fresh cilantro leaves.

Serving Suggestions: Enjoy the Ginger Carrot Soup as a warm and comforting dinner option. Serve with a slice of whole-grain bread or a side of mixed greens for a complete meal.

Turkey and Sweet Potato Hash

- **Preparation Time:** 10 minutes
- **Cooking Time:** 20 minutes
- **Serves:** 4

Ingredients:

- 1 tablespoon olive oil
- 1 lb lean ground turkey
- 2 sweet potatoes, peeled and diced
- 1 onion, diced
- 2 cloves garlic, minced
- 1 teaspoon paprika
- 1 teaspoon ground cumin
- Salt and pepper to taste

- Fresh parsley for garnish (optional)

Nutritional Information (per serving): Calories: 280 | Protein: 20g | Fat: 10g | Carbohydrates: 25g | Fiber: 4g | Sugars: 6g

Instructions:

1. In a large skillet, heat your olive oil over medium heat until warm.
2. Add lean ground turkey to the skillet and cook until browned, breaking it up with a spoon as it cooks.
3. Add diced sweet potatoes to the skillet and cook for 8-10 minutes until they start to soften.
4. Add diced onion and minced garlic to the skillet. Cook for another 3-4 minutes until the onion is translucent and fragrant.
5. Sprinkle paprika and ground cumin over the mixture in the skillet. Stir well to combine.
6. Season with salt and pepper to suit your liking.
7. Cook for an additional 5-7 minutes, stirring occasionally, until the sweet potatoes are tender and the turkey is cooked through.

8. Garnish with fresh parsley if desired.

Serving Suggestions: Serve the Turkey and Sweet Potato Hash hot, topped with a fried or poached egg if desired, for added protein and flavor. Enjoy as a satisfying dinner option on its own or with a side salad for extra freshness.

Beef and veggie Omelet

- **Preparation Time:** 10 minutes
- **Cooking Time:** 10 minutes
- **Serves:** 2

Ingredients:

- 4 large eggs
- 1/4 cup milk (or dairy-free alternative)
- 1/2 cup cooked lean beef, diced
- 1/2 cup mixed vegetables (such as bell peppers, onions, spinach), diced
- 1 tablespoon olive oil
- Salt and pepper to taste
- Fresh herbs (like chives or parsley) for garnish (optional)

Nutritional Information (per serving): Calories: 250 | Protein: 20g | Fat: 15g | Carbohydrates: 6g | Fiber: 2g | Sugars: 3g

Instructions:

1. Whisk together eggs and milk in a bowl until fully blended.
2. Season with salt and pepper according to your preference.
3. Your olive oil should be heated in a non-stick skillet over medium heat.
4. Add diced beef and mixed vegetables to the skillet. Cook for 3-4 minutes until the vegetables are tender and the beef is heated through.
5. Pour the whisked eggs over the beef and vegetables in the skillet.
6. Allow the omelet to cook undisturbed for 2-3 minutes until the edges start to set.
7. Using a spatula, gently lift the edges of the omelet and tilt the skillet to let the uncooked eggs flow underneath.

8. Once the eggs are mostly set but still slightly runny on top, sprinkle any desired herbs over the omelet.

9. Fold the omelet in half with the spatula, carefully.

10. Cook for another 1-2 minutes until the eggs are fully cooked through.

11. Slide the omelet onto a plate for serving while it's still hot.

Serving Suggestions: Serve the Beef and Veggie Omelet hot, garnished with fresh herbs if desired. Enjoy as a hearty and protein-packed dinner option, accompanied by a side salad or whole-grain toast for a balanced meal.

Salmon and Asparagus Foil Packets

- **Preparation Time:** 10 minutes
- **Cooking Time:** 20 minutes
- **Serves:** 2

Ingredients:

- 2 salmon filets
- 1 bunch asparagus, trimmed
- 1 lemon, thinly sliced

- 2 cloves garlic, minced
- 2 tablespoons olive oil
- Salt and pepper to taste
- Fresh dill for garnish (optional)

Nutritional Information (per serving): Calories: 350 | Protein: 30g | Fat: 22g | Carbohydrates: 7g | Fiber: 3g | Sugars: 2g

Instructions:

1. Preheat the oven to 400°F (200°C).
2. Cut two large pieces of aluminum foil.
3. Position a salmon filet at the center of each foil piece.
4. Arrange trimmed asparagus spears around each salmon filet.
5. Sprinkle minced garlic over the salmon and asparagus.
6. Coat the salmon and asparagus with a drizzle of olive oil.
7. Season with salt and pepper to suit your liking.
8. Place lemon slices on top of each salmon filet.

9. Fold the edges of the foil over the salmon and asparagus to create sealed packets.

10. Place the foil packets on a baking sheet and bake in the preheated oven for 15-20 minutes, or until the salmon is cooked through and flakes easily with a fork.

11. Carefully open the foil packets and transfer the salmon and asparagus to serving plates.

12. Garnish with fresh dill if desired.

Serving Suggestions:

Serve the Salmon and Asparagus Foil Packets hot, with a side of quinoa or brown rice and steamed vegetables for a nutritious and delicious dinner..

Desserts/Snacks for Afib Diet

Sugar-free Cheesecake

- **Preparation Time:** 20 minutes
- **Chilling Time:** 4 hours
- **Serves:** 8

Ingredients:

- 2 cups low-fat cottage cheese
- 8 oz reduced-fat cream cheese
- 1/2 cup plain Greek yogurt
- 1/4 cup honey or maple syrup
- 2 teaspoons vanilla extract
- 2 tablespoons cornstarch
- 2 large eggs
- 1 cup mixed berries for topping (optional)

Nutritional Information (per serving): Calories: 180 | Protein: 10g | Fat: 8g | Carbohydrates: 15g | Fiber: 1g | Sugars: 10g

Instructions:

1. Preheat the oven to 325°F (160°C). Lightly grease a 9-inch springform pan.

2. In a food processor or blender, combine cottage cheese, cream cheese, Greek yogurt, honey or maple syrup, vanilla extract, and cornstarch. Blend until smooth.

3. Add eggs to the mixture and blend until well combined.

4. Pour the mixture into the prepared springform pan and smooth the top with a spatula.

5. Bake in the preheated oven for 45-50 minutes, or until the cheesecake is firm yet slightly wobbly in the middle.

6. Turn off the oven and let the cheesecake cool slowly inside with the door ajar for around 1 hour.

7. Remove the cheesecake from the oven and refrigerate for at least 4 hours, or until completely chilled and firm.

8. Before serving, top the cheesecake with mixed berries if desired.

Serving Suggestions: Serve the Sugar-Free Cheesecake chilled, with a dollop of Greek yogurt and fresh berries for a delightful dessert or snack option.

Almond Flour Cookies

- **Preparation Time:** 15 minutes
- **Cooking Time:** 10 minutes
- **Serves:** Makes about 12 cookies

Ingredients:

- 2 cups almond flour
- 1/4 cup coconut oil, melted
- 1/4 cup honey or maple syrup
- 1 teaspoon vanilla extract
- 1/4 teaspoon baking soda
- Pinch of salt
- Optional add-ins: dark chocolate chips, chopped nuts, dried fruit

Nutritional Information (per serving, based on 1 cookie): Calories: 150 | Protein: 3g | Fat: 12g | Carbohydrates: 10g | Fiber: 2g | Sugars: 6g

Instructions:

1. Preheat the oven to 350°F (175°C). Line a baking sheet with parchment paper.

2. In a large mixing bowl, combine almond flour, melted coconut oil, honey or maple syrup, vanilla extract, baking soda, and a pinch of salt. Mix until a dough forms.

3. Add optional mix-ins like dark chocolate chips, chopped nuts, or dried fruit, and gently fold into the batter.

4. Use a cookie scoop or spoon to portion out the dough and place it onto the prepared baking sheet.

5. Use your hands or the back of a spoon to gently flatten each cookie.

6. Bake until the edges turn golden brown, typically about 8-10 minutes in the preheated oven.

7. Allow the cookies to cool on the baking sheet for a few minutes after removing them from the oven, then transfer them to a wire rack to cool completely.

Serving Suggestions: Pair with a glass of almond milk or herbal tea for a delightful treat that's perfect for satisfying cravings while adhering to an Afib diet.

Mini Veggies Frittatas

- **Preparation Time:** 15 minutes
- **Cooking Time:** 20 minutes
- **Serves:** 6

Ingredients:

- 6 large eggs
- 1/4 cup milk (or dairy-free alternative)
- 1 cup mixed vegetables (such as bell peppers, spinach, tomatoes), finely chopped
- 1/4 cup grated cheese (such as cheddar or feta)
- Salt and pepper to taste
- Cooking spray or olive oil for greasing muffin tin

Nutritional Information (per serving, based on 2 frittatas): Calories: 150 | Protein: 10g | Fat: 10g | Carbohydrates: 5g | Fiber: 1g | Sugars: 2g

Instructions:

1. Preheat the oven to 375°F (190°C). Apply cooking spray or olive oil to coat each cup of a 6-cup muffin tin.

2. In a mixing bowl, whisk eggs and milk together until evenly mixed.

3. Season with salt and pepper to suit your liking.

4. Stir in finely chopped mixed vegetables and grated cheese into the egg mixture.

5. Fill each of the greased muffin cups with an equal amount of the mixture.

6. Bake in the preheated oven for 15-20 minutes, or until the frittatas are set and lightly golden on top.

7. Remove from the oven and allow the mini frittatas to cool in the muffin tin for a few minutes.

8. Use a knife or spatula to carefully loosen the edges of the frittatas, then transfer them to a wire rack to cool completely.

Serving Suggestions: Serve alongside a side salad or whole-grain crackers for a balanced and satisfying treat.

Butternut Squash Fries

- **Preparation Time:** 15 minutes
- **Cooking Time:** 25 minutes
- **Serves:** 4

Ingredients:

- 1 medium butternut squash
- 2 tablespoons olive oil
- 1 teaspoon garlic powder
- 1 teaspoon smoked paprika
- 1/2 teaspoon salt
- 1/4 teaspoon black pepper
- Fresh parsley for garnish (optional)

Nutritional Information (per serving): Calories: 120 | Protein: 1g | Fat: 7g | Carbohydrates: 15g | Fiber: 3g | Sugars: 3g

Instructions:

1. Preheat the oven to 425°F (220°C). Line a baking sheet with parchment paper.

2. Peel the butternut squash and cut it into fries-like shapes, about 1/2-inch thick.

3. In a large bowl, toss the butternut squash fries with olive oil, garlic powder, smoked paprika, salt, and black pepper until evenly coated.

4. Arrange the seasoned butternut squash fries in a single layer on the prepared baking sheet.

5. Place the fries in the preheated oven and bake for 20-25 minutes, flipping them halfway through cooking to ensure they are evenly golden brown and crispy.

6. Remove from the oven and leave it to cool for some minutes.

7. Garnish with fresh parsley if desired.

Serving Suggestions: Enjoy these Butternut Squash Fries as a healthier alternative to traditional potato fries. Serve with a side of Greek yogurt-based dip or hummus for added flavor.

Baked Apples

- **Preparation Time:** 10 minutes
- **Cooking Time:** 30 minutes
- **Serves:** 4

Ingredients:

- 4 large apples (such as Granny Smith or Honeycrisp)
- 2 tablespoons unsalted butter, melted (or coconut oil for dairy-free option)
- 2 tablespoons honey or maple syrup
- 1 teaspoon ground cinnamon
- 1/4 cup of chopped nuts (like pecans or walnuts)
- Optional toppings: Greek yogurt, drizzle of honey, sprinkle of granola

Nutritional Information (per serving): Calories: 180 | Protein: 2g | Fat: 8g | Carbohydrates: 30g | Fiber: 5g | Sugars: 22g

Instructions:

1. Preheat the oven to 375°F (190°C). Grease your baking dish with butter or cooking spray.

2. Core the apples using an apple corer or a sharp knife, leaving the bottoms intact.

3. Place the cored apples in the prepared baking dish.

4. In a small bowl, mix together melted butter (or coconut oil), honey or maple syrup, and ground cinnamon.

5. Drizzle the honey-cinnamon mixture over the apples, ensuring they are evenly coated.

6. Spread some chopped nuts on top of each apple.

7. Wrap the baking dish with foil and place it in the preheated oven to bake for 20 minutes.

8. Take off the foil and continue baking for 10 more minutes until the apples are tender and have a golden-brown color.

9. Once done, let it cool for a few minutes before serving.

Serving Suggestions: Serve the Baked Apples warm, optionally topped with a dollop of Greek yogurt, a drizzle of honey, or a sprinkle of granola for added texture and flavor.

Beverages/Smoothies for Afib Diet

Vanilla blueberry smoothie

- **Preparation Time:** 5 minutes
- **Serves:** 2

Ingredients:

- 1 cup fresh or frozen blueberries
- 1 ripe banana
- 1/2 cup plain Greek yogurt
- 1/2 cup unsweetened almond milk (or any milk of choice)
- 1 teaspoon pure vanilla extract
- 1 tablespoon maple syrup or honey (optional, adjust to taste)
- Ice cubes (optional)

Nutritional Information (per serving): Calories: 150 | Protein: 6g | Fat: 1g | Carbohydrates: 30g | Fiber: 4g | Sugars: 20g

Instructions:

1. In a blender, combine blueberries, bananas, Greek yogurt, almond milk, vanilla extract, and honey or maple syrup (if using).

2. Keep blending until the mixture reaches a smooth and creamy consistency, adding ice cubes if you want it colder.
3. Taste and adjust sweetness with additional honey or maple syrup if needed.
4. Pour into glasses and serve immediately.

Serving Suggestions: Pair with a handful of nuts for added protein and healthy fats.

Moocha Banana Smoothie

- **Preparation Time:** 5 minutes
- **Serves:** 2

Ingredients:

- 1 ripe banana
- 1 cup brewed coffee, cooled
- 1/2 cup plain Greek yogurt
- 1 tablespoon unsweetened cocoa powder
- 1 tablespoon maple syrup or honey (optional, adjust to taste)
- Ice cubes (optional)

Nutritional Information (per serving): Calories: 120 | Protein: 6g | Fat: 1g | Carbohydrates: 24g | Fiber: 3g | Sugars: 14g

Instructions:

1. In a blender, combine ripe banana, brewed coffee, Greek yogurt, unsweetened cocoa powder, and honey or maple syrup (if using).
2. Blend until smooth and creamy.
3. Add ice cubes if a colder consistency is desired, and blend again until smooth.
4. Taste and adjust sweetness with additional honey or maple syrup if needed.
5. Pour into glasses and serve immediately.

Serving Suggestions:

Pair with a sprinkle of cocoa nibs or a dollop of whipped cream for an extra indulgent treat.

Ginger Tea

- **Preparation Time:** 10 minutes
- **Serves:** 2

Ingredients:

- 2 cups water
- 2 teaspoons fresh ginger, grated or sliced
- 1 tablespoon honey (optional)
- Lemon slices for garnish (optional)

Nutritional Information (per serving): Calories: 10 | Protein: 0g | Fat: 0g | Carbohydrates: 3g | Fiber: 0g | Sugars: 3g

Instructions:

1. Heat water in a saucepan until it reaches a boiling point.
2. Add grated or sliced ginger to the boiling water.
3. Reduce the heat to low and let the ginger simmer for 5-7 minutes.

4. Remove the saucepan from heat and let the ginger steep in the hot water for an additional 5 minutes.
5. Strain the ginger tea into cups using a fine mesh sieve or tea strainer.
6. Stir in honey to taste, if desired.
7. Garnish with lemon slices, if using.
8. Serve hot.

Serving Suggestions: Enjoy Ginger Tea as a soothing and warming beverage option, perfect for relaxation or to help alleviate digestive discomfort. Sip slowly and savor the spicy yet refreshing flavor of ginger.

Warm Turmeric Milk

- **Preparation Time:** 5 minutes
- **Cooking Time:** 5 minutes
- **Serves:** 2

Ingredients:
- 2 cups milk (dairy or plant-based)
- 1 teaspoon ground turmeric

- 1/2 teaspoon ground cinnamon
- 1/4 teaspoon ground ginger
- 1 tablespoon maple syrup or honey (optional, adjust to taste)
- Pinch of black pepper (optional)

Nutritional Information (per serving): Calories: 120 | Protein: 8g | Fat: 5g | Carbohydrates: 12g | Fiber: 1g | Sugars: 10g

Instructions:

1. In a small saucepan, heat the milk over medium-low heat until warmed through, but not boiling.
2. Stir in ground turmeric, ground cinnamon, and ground ginger.
3. Add honey or maple syrup to sweeten, if desired, and stir until dissolved.
4. If using, add a pinch of black pepper, as it helps enhance the absorption of curcumin, the active compound in turmeric.

5. Continue to heat the mixture for another 2-3 minutes, stirring occasionally, until fragrant and well combined.
6. Remove from heat and pour the warm turmeric milk into cups.
7. Serve immediately.

Serving Suggestions: Sprinkle a dash of ground cinnamon on top for extra flavor and aroma.

Vegetable Juice

- **Preparation Time:** 10 minutes
- **Serves:** 2

Ingredients:

- 2 large carrots
- 2 stalks celery
- 1 cucumber
- 1 beetroot, peeled
- 1 small piece of ginger (about 1 inch)
- 1 lemon, peeled
- Optional: handful of spinach or kale for added greens

Nutritional Information (per serving): Calories: 70 | Protein: 2g | Fat: 0g | Carbohydrates: 17g | Fiber: 5g | Sugars: 10g

Instructions:

1. Wash and prepare all vegetables and fruit by chopping them into smaller pieces as needed to fit into your juicer chute.
2. Pass all the vegetables and fruit through a juicer according to its instructions, extracting the juice.
3. Once all the ingredients have been juiced, stir the mixture to combine.
4. If desired, strain the juice through a fine mesh sieve or cheesecloth to remove any pulp.
5. Pour the vegetable juice into glasses.
6. Serve immediately over ice, if desired, or refrigerate until chilled before serving.

Serving Suggestions: Enjoy Vegetable Juice as a refreshing and nutritious beverage option, packed with vitamins, minerals, and antioxidants from a variety of colorful vegetables and fruits.

CHAPTER 3

30-Day Meal Plan Sample for Afib Diet

Please note that the provided meal plan is a sample and should not be interpreted as a recommendation to consume all the listed recipes in a single day.

This meal plan aims to offer inspiration and guidance for healthy meal preparation. Feel free to customize this plan to suit your preferences and dietary requirements. Adjust portions and ingredients based on individual preferences and dietary needs.

Day 1:
- Breakfast: Peanut Butter-Banana Cinnamon Toast
- Lunch: Soft Scrambled Tofu with Veggies
- Dinner: Mexican Platter
- Dessert/Snack: Sugar-Free Cheesecake
- Beverage: Vanilla Blueberry Smoothie

Day 2:
- Breakfast: Mango-Almond Smoothie Bowl

- Lunch: Garlic Mashed Cauliflower
- Dinner: Lemon Rosemary Chicken
- Dessert/Snack: Almond Flour Cookies
- Beverage: Mocha Banana Smoothie

Day 3:

- Breakfast: Vegan Breakfast Burrito
- Lunch: Spring Vegetable Stir-Fried Rice
- Dinner: Rainbow Collard Wraps
- Dessert/Snack: Mini Veggie Frittatas
- Beverage: Ginger Tea

Day 4:

- Breakfast: Almond Flour Banana Bread
- Lunch: Easy Tofu Fajitas
- Dinner: Ginger Carrot Soup
- Dessert/Snack: Butternut Squash Fries
- Beverage: Warm Turmeric Milk

Day 5:

- Breakfast: Mediterranean Breakfast Salad
- Lunch: Colorful Veggie Stew with Turkey Tenders

- Dinner: Beef and Veggie Omelette
- Dessert/Snack: Baked Apples
- Beverage: Vegetable Juice

Day 6:

- Breakfast: Creamy Blueberry-Pecan Oatmeal
- Lunch: Raw Vegan Gazpacho
- Dinner: Salmon and Asparagus Foil Packets
- Dessert/Snack: Banana Nut Pancakes
- Beverage: Ginger Tea

Day 7:

- Breakfast: Breakfast Porridge
- Lunch: Soft Scrambled Tofu with Veggies
- Dinner: Egg Drop Soup
- Dessert/Snack: Mediterranean Breakfast Salad (variation with extra nuts and fruits)
- Beverage: Vanilla Blueberry Smoothie

Day 8:

- Breakfast: Mango-Almond Smoothie Bowl
- Lunch: Garlic Mashed Cauliflower
- Dinner: Lemon Rosemary Chicken
- Dessert/Snack: Sugar-Free Cheesecake

- Beverage: Mocha Banana Smoothie

Day 9:
- Breakfast: Vegan Breakfast Burrito
- Lunch: Spring Vegetable Stir-Fried Rice
- Dinner: Rainbow Collard Wraps
- Dessert/Snack: Almond Flour Cookies
- Beverage: Ginger Tea

Day 10:
- Breakfast: Almond Flour Banana Bread
- Lunch: Easy Tofu Fajitas
- Dinner: Ginger Carrot Soup
- Dessert/Snack: Butternut Squash Fries
- Beverage: Warm Turmeric Milk

Day 11:
- Breakfast: Mediterranean Breakfast Salad
- Lunch: Colorful Veggie Stew with Turkey Tenders
- Dinner: Beef and Veggie Omelette
- Dessert/Snack: Baked Apples
- Beverage: Vegetable Juice

Day 12:

- Breakfast: Creamy Blueberry-Pecan Oatmeal
- Lunch: Raw Vegan Gazpacho
- Dinner: Salmon and Asparagus Foil Packets
- Dessert/Snack: Banana Nut Pancakes
- Beverage: Ginger Tea

Day 13:
- Breakfast: Breakfast Porridge
- Lunch: Soft Scrambled Tofu with Veggies
- Dinner: Egg Drop Soup
- Dessert/Snack: Mediterranean Breakfast Salad (variation with extra nuts and fruits)
- Beverage: Vanilla Blueberry Smoothie

Day 14:
- Breakfast: Peanut Butter-Banana Cinnamon Toast
- Lunch: Garlic Mashed Cauliflower
- Dinner: Mexican Platter
- Dessert/Snack: Sugar-Free Cheesecake
- Beverage: Mocha Banana Smoothie

Day 15:

- Breakfast: Vegan Breakfast Burrito
- Lunch: Lemon Rosemary Chicken
- Dinner: Salmon and Asparagus Foil Packets
- Dessert/Snack: Almond Flour Cookies
- Beverage: Ginger Tea

Day 16:

- Breakfast: Creamy Blueberry-Pecan Oatmeal
- Lunch: Colorful Veggie Stew with Turkey Tenders
- Dinner: Beef and Veggie Omelette
- Dessert/Snack: Mini Veggie Frittatas
- Beverage: Vanilla Blueberry Smoothie

Day 17:

- Breakfast: Banana Nut Pancakes
- Lunch: Raw Vegan Gazpacho
- Dinner: Mexican Platter
- Dessert/Snack: Sugar-Free Cheesecake
- Beverage: Mocha Banana Smoothie

Day 18:

- Breakfast: Breakfast Porridge
- Lunch: Soft Scrambled Tofu with Veggies
- Dinner: Egg Drop Soup
- Dessert/Snack: Baked Apples
- Beverage: Warm Turmeric Milk

Day 19:

- Breakfast: Mango-Almond Smoothie Bowl
- Lunch: Garlic Mashed Cauliflower
- Dinner: Rainbow Collard Wraps
- Dessert/Snack: Butternut Squash Fries
- Beverage: Vegetable Juice

Day 20:

- Breakfast: Almond Flour Banana Bread
- Lunch: Spring Vegetable Stir-Fried Rice
- Dinner: Ginger Carrot Soup
- Dessert/Snack: Mini Veggies Frittatas
- Beverage: Ginger Tea

Day 21:

- Breakfast: Mediterranean Breakfast Salad

- Lunch: Easy Tofu Fajitas
- Dinner: Turkey and Sweet Potato Hash
- Dessert/Snack: Almond Flour Cookies
- Beverage: Vanilla Blueberry Smoothie

Day 22:

- Breakfast: Creamy Blueberry-Pecan Oatmeal
- Lunch: Colorful Veggie Stew with Turkey Tenders
- Dinner: Beef and Veggie Omelette
- Dessert/Snack: Sugar-Free Cheesecake
- Beverage: Mocha Banana Smoothie

Day 23:

- Breakfast: Banana Nut Pancakes
- Lunch: Raw Vegan Gazpacho
- Dinner: Salmon and Asparagus Foil Packets
- Dessert/Snack: Baked Apples
- Beverage: Warm Turmeric Milk

Day 24:

- Breakfast: Breakfast Porridge
- Lunch: Soft Scrambled Tofu with Veggies
- Dinner: Egg Drop Soup
- Dessert/Snack: Butternut Squash Fries

- Beverage: Vegetable Juice

Day 25:

- Breakfast: Mango-Almond Smoothie Bowl
- Lunch: Garlic Mashed Cauliflower
- Dinner: Rainbow Collard Wraps
- Dessert/Snack: Mini Veggie Frittatas
- Beverage: Ginger Tea

Day 26:

- Breakfast: Almond Flour Banana Bread
- Lunch: Spring Vegetable Stir-Fried Rice
- Dinner: Ginger Carrot Soup
- Dessert/Snack: Sugar-Free Cheesecake
- Beverage: Vanilla Blueberry Smoothie

Day 27:

- Breakfast: Mediterranean Breakfast Salad
- Lunch: Easy Tofu Fajitas
- Dinner: Turkey and Sweet Potato Hash
- Dessert/Snack: Almond Flour Cookies
- Beverage: Mocha Banana Smoothie

Day 28:

- Breakfast: Creamy Blueberry-Pecan Oatmeal
- Lunch: Colorful Veggie Stew with Turkey Tenders
- Dinner: Beef and Veggie Omelette
- Dessert/Snack: Baked Apples
- Beverage: Warm Turmeric Milk

Day 29:

- Breakfast: Banana Nut Pancakes
- Lunch: Raw Vegan Gazpacho
- Dinner: Salmon and Asparagus Foil Packets
- Dessert/Snack: Butternut Squash Fries
- Beverage: Vegetable Juice

Day 30:

- Breakfast: Breakfast Porridge
- Lunch: Soft Scrambled Tofu with Veggies
- Dinner: Egg Drop Soup
- Dessert/Snack: Mini Veggies Frittatas
- Beverage: Ginger Tea

CHAPTER 4

Conclusion

As we wrap up this book, I want to leave you with this: your journey to better heart health starts here. By embracing the principles of the Afib diet and incorporating the delicious recipes provided in this book into your daily routine, you're taking proactive steps towards a healthier you.

But remember, this isn't just about following a set of rules—it's about nourishing your body and embracing a lifestyle that supports your well-being. So as you dive into these recipes, I encourage you to savor the flavors, get creative in the kitchen, and make each meal a celebration of good health.

And while this cookbook is a great starting point, your journey doesn't end here. Keep exploring, keep learning, and keep listening to your body. Ultimately, it's about finding what works best for you and making sustainable changes that you can stick with for the long haul.

Here's to your wellness and vitality. May your meals be delicious, your heart be happy, and your journey towards wellness be filled with joy and abundance. Thank you for joining me on this adventure, and cheers to a lifetime of good eating and good health!

Made in the USA
Las Vegas, NV
22 July 2024

92720694R00052